The Comprehensive Anti Inflammatory Guide and Cookbook for Beginners

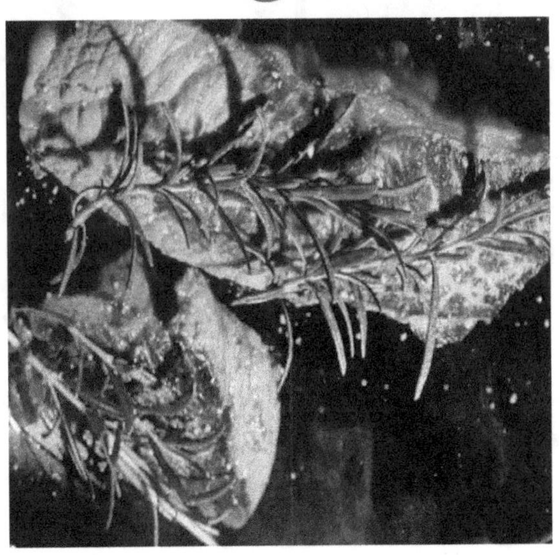

Lose weight, detoxify your body, and restore well-being with the Anti-Inflammatory Diet through 52 weeks of quick, simple home made recipes.

Dr.Raymond Harris

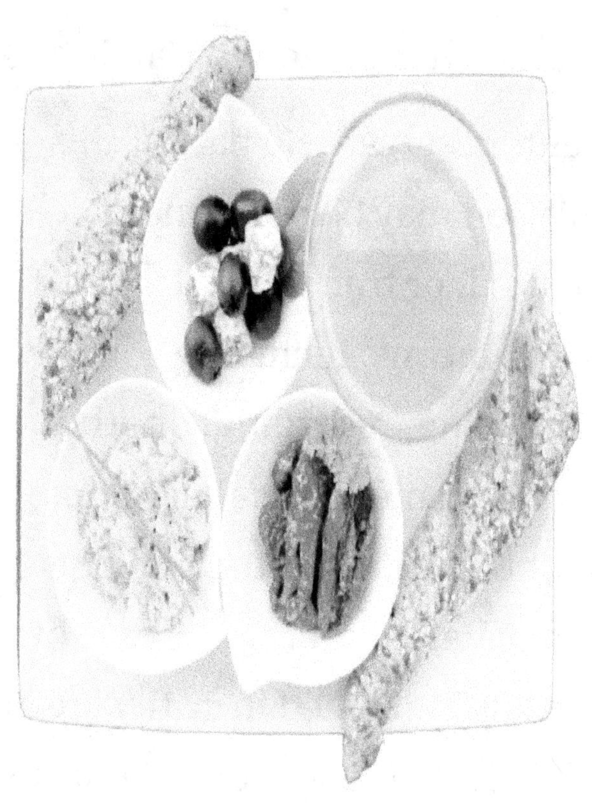

Table of content

INTRODUCTION

A basic biological reaction, inflammation is an essential component of the body's defensive systems and plays a vital part in their process. Inflammation is the body's means of defending itself against potentially damaging stimuli, such as viruses, irritants, or damaged cells. At its foundation, inflammation is a defense mechanism.

Chronic inflammation may have negative consequences on the body, leading to a variety of illnesses and ailments, despite the fact that this process is necessary for the maintenance of general health.

First and foremost, it is necessary to acknowledge the dual character of inflammation, which may be either acute or chronic.

An acute inflammation is a quick and localized reaction that occurs in the body in response to an injury or illness. Through the release of immune cells, hormones, and nutrients to the afflicted region, it kickstarts the healing process and helps the body recover from the injury.

As an example, consider the redness and swelling that surround a cut, as well as the warmth that is linked with an infection. In this approach, the body is able to isolate and heal any harm that has occurred.

On the other hand, chronic inflammation is a continual, low-grade reaction that continues over a protracted time. Chronic inflammation, on the other hand, may have an effect on the whole body, in contrast to acute inflammation, which is a protective and confined reaction. It is often a covert and sneaky force that may go undiscovered for a considerable amount of time. Factors such as a sedentary lifestyle, poor food, stress, and environmental pollutants may contribute to the development of chronic inflammation.
The significance of diagnosing and managing chronic inflammation cannot be emphasized.

Research has linked chronic inflammation to a range of health conditions, including cardiovascular illnesses, diabetes, autoimmune disorders, and even some malignancies. By understanding the causes underlying inflammation, people may make educated decisions to limit its influence on their health. This gets us to the notion of an anti-inflammatory diet – a significant tool in controlling and avoiding chronic inflammation. An anti-inflammatory diet focuses on ingesting foods that assist control the body's inflammatory response while avoiding those that may increase it.

Key components of such a diet include whole foods rich in antioxidants, omega-3 fatty acids, and phytonutrients.

The association between nutrition and inflammation is deep and varied. Certain foods, such as berries, leafy greens, and fatty fish, exhibit anti-inflammatory qualities, helping to reduce the inflammatory response. In contrast, a diet strong in processed foods, refined carbohydrates, and saturated fats may cause inflammation. Recognizing these dietary impacts helps people to make decisions that favorably improve their inflammatory balance.

Beyond its direct effect on physical health, inflammation also profoundly impacts mental well-being. Emerging evidence reveals a substantial association between chronic inflammation and mental health issues, including sadness and anxiety. Understanding this relationship stresses the holistic aspect of health and encourages people to embrace lifestyle choices that improve both physical and mental well-being.

As we dive into the subtleties of how inflammation impacts health, it becomes obvious that this physiological process is not isolated to a certain system or organ. Rather, it pervades every facet of our well-being, serving as a quiet orchestrator in the backdrop of our everyday lives. From joint discomfort to digestive difficulties, the signs of chronic inflammation may be broad and extensive.

In the next chapters of this thorough guide and cookbook, we will examine the fundamentals of an anti-inflammatory lifestyle. We will begin on a journey through the fundamentals of anti-inflammatory diet, uncovering the power of whole foods, maximizing protein choices, and unlocking the potential of herbs and spices. Additionally, we will go into the areas of detoxification, weight control, and mindful eating, acknowledging the interconnectivity of these factors in nurturing total health.

By obtaining insights into the complicated dance between inflammation and our bodies, we empower ourselves with the information required to make mindful decisions that enhance well-being. This book intends to be a companion on

your route to knowledge, giving
practical suggestions, tasty recipes,
and a comprehensive approach to
adopting an anti-inflammatory
lifestyle. As we traverse the
complicated terrain of health, let us go
on this adventure together,
empowered to make choices that
resonate with vitality and longevity.

Chapter one

Weeks 1-4: Building the Foundation

Embarking on a road toward an anti-inflammatory lifestyle starts with having a firm foundation. These early weeks are key for building the framework, knowing the principles of anti-inflammatory food, filling your cupboard with staples, and mastering easy meal preparation skills. Let's go into each of these components to set the foundation for a revolutionary and sustainable lifestyle.

Basics of Anti-Inflammatory Eating
Anti-inflammatory eating is not a restricted diet but a comprehensive approach that stresses entire, nutrient-dense meals. At its foundation, it tries to regulate the body's inflammatory response by integrating foods that promote health and avoiding those that contribute to inflammation.

1. Embrace Colorful, Whole Foods: Include a variety of fruits and vegetables in your diet, striving for a rainbow of hues. These plant-based meals are rich in vitamins, minerals, and antioxidants that reduce inflammation.

2. Prioritize Omega-3 Fatty Acids: Incorporate sources of omega-3 fatty acids, such as fatty fish (salmon, mackerel), flaxseeds, chia seeds, and walnuts. These essential fats have anti-inflammatory qualities and improve general well-being.

3. Choose Whole Grains: Opt for whole grains like quinoa, brown rice, and oats instead of processed grains. Whole grains include fiber and minerals that help to a healthy gut and prevent inflammation.

4. Include Lean Proteins: Select lean protein sources such chicken, beans, lentils, and tofu.

Protein is vital for tissue repair and immunological function, and selecting lean choices helps maintain a healthy balance.

5. Healthy Fats Are Key:
   Incorporate sources of healthy fats, such as avocado, olive oil, and almonds. These fats not only produce a sensation of fullness but also have anti-inflammatory properties.

6. Mindful Hydration: Stay hydrated with water, herbal teas, and infusions. Proper hydration is vital for general health and promotes the body's natural detoxifying processes.

Understanding these core concepts lays the groundwork for making educated dietary choices that match with an anti-inflammatory lifestyle.

 Pantry Essentials

A well-stocked pantry is the backbone of efficient meal planning and preparation. Ensuring you have crucial components easily accessible simplifies the cooking process and promotes the adoption of anti-inflammatory foods into your everyday meals. Here's a guide to important pantry items:

1. Whole Grains: Brown rice, quinoa, oats, and whole wheat pasta offer the basis for healthful meals.

2. Legumes: Stock up on canned or dry beans, lentils, and chickpeas. These are flexible, protein-rich mainstays.

3. Healthy Oils: Olive oil, avocado oil, and coconut oil are good alternatives for cooking and dressing salads, offering healthy fats.

4. Herbs and Spices: Build a collection of anti-inflammatory herbs and spices like turmeric, ginger, garlic, and cinnamon to boost taste and health benefits.

5. Nuts and Seeds: Almonds, walnuts, flaxseeds, and chia seeds are fantastic for snacking and providing nutritious value to meals.

6. Canned Tomatoes: Tomatoes are a versatile component for sauces, stews, and soups. Choose canned tomatoes without additional sugars.

7. Lean Proteins: Stock your freezer with lean proteins like chicken breast, fish fillets, and tofu for easy and healthful dinner alternatives.

8. Whole Food Sweeteners: Opt for natural sweeteners like honey or maple syrup instead of processed sugars.

9. Non-Dairy Alternatives: Explore non-dairy milk choices such as almond, coconut, or oat milk for a dairy-free alternative.

10. Whole-Grain snacking: Keep whole-grain crackers, rice cakes, or popcorn on hand for fast and tasty snacking.

Having these items on hand makes it easy to construct healthful meals that correspond with your anti-inflammatory aims.

Simple Meal Prep Tips

Efficient meal preparation is a cornerstone of keeping a regular and pleasurable anti-inflammatory diet. Here are practical strategies to improve your meal prep process:

1. Plan Your Meals: Take time each week to plan your meals, considering a mix of meats, veggies, and healthy grains. This helps minimize impulsive and perhaps less nutritious meal choices.

2. Batch Cooking: Prepare bigger amounts of essentials like grains, beans, or roasted vegetables to utilize throughout the week. This saves time and ensures you have components readily accessible for making meals.

3. Pre-cut Vegetables and Fruits: Wash, peel, and chop vegetables and fruits in advance. Having these ready-to-go components promotes healthy snacking and allows speedier meal assembling.

4. Marinate Proteins: Marinate proteins in advance with aromatic herbs and spices. This not only improves the flavor but also decreases cooking time when it's time to make the dish.

5. Use Mason Jar Salads: Assemble salads in mason jars, beginning with the dressing at the bottom and adding sturdier items first.

This keeps the salad fresh and crisp
until you're ready to eat it.

6. Freeze Individual Portions
   Portion and freeze soups, stews, or
casseroles for days when you have less
time to prepare. This avoids
dependence on less healthy
convenience alternatives.

7. Invest in Storage Containers: –
Purchase a variety of storage containers
to keep your ready goods and meals
organized. Glass containers are a
fantastic eco-friendly alternative.

8. Explore One-Pan dishes: Simplify clean-up and save time by creating dishes that can be prepared on a single pan. Sheet pan meals or one-pot dishes are easy and flexible.

9. Keep Snacks Ready: - Prepare grab-and-go snacks like pre-portioned almonds, cut veggies, or fruit to alleviate hunger between meals.

10. Stay Flexible: While meal planning is essential, allow for flexibility. Life may be unexpected, so keeping a few fast and healthy meals on hand means you can adjust to changing situations.

Building the basis for an anti-inflammatory lifestyle entails not only comprehending the concepts of healthy eating but also practical execution via a well-stocked pantry and quick meal preparation. These early weeks serve as a springboard for the transformational journey ahead, bringing you toward sustainable well-being and energy. As we go ahead, let's continue examining the different dimensions of anti-inflammatory living, revealing the richness that comes from supporting our bodies with purpose and care.

Chapter two

Weeks 5-12: The Power of Whole Foods

Incorporating Fruits and Vegetables

Fruits and vegetables constitute the cornerstone of an anti-inflammatory diet, supplying a wealth of vitamins, minerals, fiber, and antioxidants. Incorporating a range of colors and varieties provides a wide assortment of nutrients.

Let's examine practical methods to make fruits and veggies a vivid part of your everyday meals:

1. Rainbow Plate Approach: Aim for a colorful plate by incorporating a range of fruits and vegetables. Different hues generally represent unique nutrients, and this variety adds to overall health.

2. Seasonal Choices: Embrace seasonal food to experience optimum freshness and taste. Seasonal fruits and vegetables are not only more economical but also help local agriculture.

3. Raw and Cooked Varieties: Balance
between raw and cooked types of fruits
and vegetables. While raw choices
retain more enzymes and minerals,
heating may boost the bioavailability of
some components.

4. Smoothies and Juices: Blend fruits
and vegetables into smoothies or
produce pleasant juices. This is a
fantastic approach to enhance your
consumption, particularly if you find it
tough to consume them in their entire
form.

5. Snack Smart: Replace processed snacks with fresh fruit or vegetable snacks. Sliced cucumbers, carrot sticks, or apple slices with nut butter are delightful and healthful alternatives.

6. Incorporate Leafy Greens: Make leafy greens a mainstay in your diet. Spinach, kale, and Swiss chard are rich in vitamins and minerals. They may be added to salads, soups, or sautéed as a side dish.

7. Dress with Herbs: Enhance the taste of salads and meals with fresh herbs. Herbs like basil, cilantro, and parsley

not only enhance flavor but also give antioxidants.

8. Explore new Varieties: Step out of your comfort zone and sample new fruits and veggies. This adds excitement to your meals and brings new nutrients to your diet.

By incorporating fruits and vegetables creatively into your meals, you not only enhance your anti-inflammatory consumption but also create a visually pleasing and gratifying gastronomic experience.

Exploring Whole Grains

Whole grains are an important component of an anti-inflammatory diet, supplying fiber, vitamins, and minerals. They contribute to a steady blood sugar level and assist intestinal health. Here's how to discover the world of whole grains:

1. Diversify Your Choices: - Include a range of whole grains such as quinoa, brown rice, oats, barley, and farro. Each adds a distinct collection of nutrients to the table.

2. Swap Refined Grains: Replace refined grains with their full equivalents. Choose whole-grain

bread, pasta, and cereal to improve the nutritious value of your meals.

3. Experiment with Ancient Grains:

Try ancient grains like amaranth, freekeh, or teff. These grains have diverse tastes and nutritional qualities, adding dimension to your recipes.

4. Make Grains the Base: Build meals around healthful grains. Create grain bowls with a variety of veggies, lean meats, and tasty dressings for a filling and healthy supper.

5. Grains in Breakfast: Incorporate entire grains throughout your breakfast. Opt for oatmeal, whole grain cereal, or quinoa porridge to launch your day with prolonged energy.

6. Homemade Baked Goods: Experiment with baking with whole grain flours. Whole wheat flour, almond flour, or coconut flour may be fantastic alternatives in recipes for muffins, pancakes, or bread.

7. Balance Portion Sizes: While whole grains are healthful, balance is crucial. Pay attention to portion proportions to maintain a well-rounded diet.

Nuts, Seeds, and Healthy Fats

Healthy fats serve a critical part in an anti-inflammatory diet, contributing to heart health and general well-being. Nuts and seeds are significant sources of these healthy fats, along with critical minerals. Here's how to make them a joyful part of your everyday meals:

1. Snack on Nuts: Replace manufactured snacks with a handful of nuts. Almonds, walnuts, and pistachios give a delightful crunch while supplying heart-healthy fats.

2. Sprinkle Seeds: Add seeds like chia, flax, pumpkin, and sunflower to your meals. Sprinkle them over yogurt, salads, or include them into smoothies for an extra nutritious boost.

3. Include Avocado: - Avocado is a diverse and nutrient-dense source of healthful fats. Spread it on toast, add it to salads, or enjoy it in smoothies.

4. Choose Healthy Oils: Cook using oils high in monounsaturated fats, such as olive oil and avocado oil. These oils not only add taste to your foods but also give anti-inflammatory effects.

5. Fatty Fish: Include fatty fish like
salmon, mackerel, and trout in your
diet. These fish are rich in omega-3
fatty acids, recognized for their
anti-inflammatory qualities

6. Homemade Trail Mix:
Create your own trail mix with a variety
of nuts, seeds, and dried fruits. It
makes for easy and healthful snack.

7. Nut Butters:
Opt for pure nut butters without
additional sweeteners or oils. Spread
them over whole-grain bread, add

them to smoothies, or use them as a
dip for fresh fruit.

By combining these whole foods into
your regular meals, you not only
increase the taste and texture of your
dishes but also maximize your
nutritional intake. These weeks serve
as a trip into the vast and delightful
world of anti-inflammatory food,
offering a strong basis for prolonged
well-being. As we continue to
investigate, let's relish in the richness
of entire foods and the beneficial
influence they bring to our bodies and
lives.

Weeks 13-26: Protein-Rich Options

Lean Protein Choices

Protein is an essential component of a well-rounded anti-inflammatory diet, contributing to muscular strength, immunological function, and general vitality. Opting for lean protein sources ensures that you obtain these advantages without additional saturated fats. Let's examine a range of lean protein alternatives to vary your meals and enhance your health.

1. Poultry:
Choose lean cuts of poultry, such as skinless chicken breast or turkey.

These alternatives deliver high-quality protein without excessive saturated fats.

2. Fish:
Fatty fish like salmon, mackerel, and trout are not only rich in omega-3 fatty acids but also deliver a large protein increase. Grilling or baking fish boosts its taste without losing nutritional value.

3. Lean Cuts of Meat:
Select thin cuts of beef or pig, such as sirloin or loin. Trimming visible fat before cooking and selecting for cooking techniques like grilling or roasting further minimizes fat content.

4. Eggs:
Eggs are a diverse and complete protein source. Whether boiled, poached, or scrambled, they are a practical alternative for breakfast or a quick snack.

5. Greek Yogurt:
Greek yogurt is not only high in protein but also delivers helpful probiotics. Choose basic, unsweetened varieties and add your own fruits or nuts for taste.

6. Cottage Cheese:
Cottage cheese is another dairy alternative strong in protein.

It may be consumed on its own or added to salads, smoothies, or fruit bowls.

7. Legumes:
Incorporate legumes like lentils, chickpeas, and black beans into your meals. These plant-based sources are not only high in protein but also supply fiber and numerous vitamins.

8. Tofu with Tempeh:
Tofu and tempeh are good plant-based protein choices. They absorb flavors well and may be used in a number of cuisines, from stir-fries to salads.

9. Lean Deli Meats:
If you choose for deli meats, consider lean choices such as turkey or chicken breast. Look for products without additional preservatives or excessive sodium.

10. Seafood:
Explore a range of seafood alternatives including shrimp, scallops, and white fish. These alternatives are not only high in protein but also low in saturated fats.

Diversifying your protein sources with lean choices not only satisfies your

nutritional requirements but also
provides excitement and diversity to
your meals.

Plant-Based Proteins

Plant-based proteins provide a
plethora of minerals, fiber, and
antioxidants, making them vital to an
anti-inflammatory diet. Whether
you're following a vegetarian or just
wanting to integrate more plant-based
meals, there are various protein-rich
choices to investigate.

1. Quinoa:
Quinoa is a complete protein,
delivering all necessary amino acids.
It's a versatile grain that may be used as
a foundation for salads, bowls, or side
dishes.

2. Chia Seeds:
Chia seeds are not only high in protein
but also rich in omega-3 fatty acids and
fiber. Add them to smoothies, yogurt,
or make chia seed puddings for a
healthy boost.

3. Lentils:
Lentils are a protein and fiber
powerhouse. They may be used in

soups, stews, salads, or as a meat alternative in many cuisines.

4. Chickpeas:
Chickpeas, whether roasted for a snack, mixed into hummus, or added to curries and salads, are a great plant-based protein source.

5. Edamame:
- Edamame, or young soybeans, are high in protein and make for a pleasant snack. They may also be added to salads or consumed as a side dish.

6. Nuts:
Almonds, walnuts, and pistachios are

not only tasty but also rich in protein. They make for a simple and portable snack.

7. Seitan:
 Seitan, manufactured from wheat gluten, is a versatile and protein-rich meat alternative. It absorbs tastes effectively, making it excellent for a range of cuisines.

8. Tofu with Tempeh:
Tofu and tempeh, made from soybeans, are mainstays in plant-based diets. They may be marinated and used in stir-fries, salads, or sandwiches.

9. Plant-Based Protein Powder:
Consider adding plant-based protein powder to smoothies or dishes. Options like pea protein, hemp protein, or brown rice protein give a simple boost.

10. Spirulina:
Spirulina, a nutrient-dense algae, is not only a source of protein but also includes important vitamins and minerals. Add it to smoothies or integrate it into energy snacks.

Integrating plant-based proteins into your meals not only diversifies your nutritional intake but also corresponds with sustainable and ecologically responsible food choices.

Chapter three

Cooking Techniques for Optimal Nutrition

The manner you cook your meals might alter the nutritional composition of the components. Employing cooking procedures that keep the integrity of nutrients guarantees that you obtain the greatest value from your meal. Here are culinary ideas for maximum nutrition:

1. Steaming:
Steaming veggies helps retain their color, texture,

and nutritional content. It's a moderate cooking procedure that maintains water-soluble vitamins like vitamin C.

2. Sautéing:

Sautéing with a small quantity of oil maintains the taste and nutrients of veggies. Use heart-healthy oils like olive oil for an extra nutritional boost.

3. Grilling:

Grilling is a tasty process that provides a smokey taste to your meal. It's especially appropriate for lean meats, fish, and vegetables. Marinate proteins in herbs and spices for extra anti-inflammatory properties.

4. Baking and Roasting:
Baking and roasting vegetables and meats caramelizes their natural sugars and enriches tastes without extra additional oil. It's a flexible method for a range of components

5. Poaching:
Poaching is a delicate cooking procedure, frequently used for fish and eggs. It preserves moisture and is appropriate for sensitive proteins.

6. Pressure Cooking:
Pressure cooking maintains nutrients in food by shortening cooking time. It's an efficient way for lentils, cereals, and harder portions of meat.

7. Blanching:
Blanching involves short cooking vegetables and then instantly chilling them in cold water. This helps keep their brilliant color and nutritious richness.

8. Raw Preparations:
Enjoying various fruits and vegetables uncooked guarantees that you acquire their optimum nutritious advantages. Add raw ingredients to salads, snacks, or as garnishes.

9. Homemade Broths:
Prepare homemade broths for soups and stews using nutrient-rich

ingredients. This improves the taste of your foods while giving extra health advantages.

10. Limiting High-Temperature Frying:
While occasional frying may be part of a balanced diet, it's vital to minimize high-temperature frying since it may lead to the creation of hazardous chemicals. Choose healthier cooking techniques for frequent usage.

Understanding and executing these cooking methods not only helps to the overall nutritional content of your meals but also provides diversity and taste to your anti-inflammatory journey.

11. Herbs and Spices:
Enhance the taste of your food using herbs and spices instead of excessive salt or sugar. Not only do they contribute flavor, but many herbs and spices also come with their own anti-inflammatory effects.

12. Mindful Portioning:
Be aware of portion amounts to prevent overeating. Proper portion management not only promotes a

balanced diet but also helps maintain a healthy weight, which is vital for general well-being.

13. Combining Complementary Proteins:
For individuals following a plant-based diet, mixing complementary proteins (such as beans and grains) offers a well-rounded amino acid profile. This technique boosts the nutritional quality of your meals.

14. Marinating Proteins:
Marinating meats before cooking not only enhances taste but might also have significant health advantages.

Ingredients like olive oil, garlic, and
herbs in marinades may add to
anti-inflammatory benefits.

15. Choose Whole Foods:
Opt for whole, less processed meals
wherever feasible. Whole foods retain
more of their inherent nutrients and
fiber compared to overly processed
substitutes.

16. Heritage and Local Varieties:
Explore historical and local types of
grains, vegetables, and fruits. These
kinds generally feature distinct
nutritional profiles and may offer
variety to your diet.

17. Potate Protein Sources:
Rotate your protein sources throughout
the week. This not only reduces dietary
monotony but also assures a greater
spectrum of nutrients.

18. Homemade Dressings and Sauces:
Create homemade dressings and sauces
using heart-healthy oils, herbs, and
spices. This enables you to regulate the
contents and eliminate extra sweets or
bad fats.

19. Incorporate Fermented Foods:
Include fermented foods like yogurt,
kimchi, or sauerkraut in your diet.

These foods are high in probiotics, which boost gut health and general immunological function.

20. Practice Mindful Eating:
Practice mindful eating by savoring each mouthful, paying attention to hunger and fullness indicators, and enjoying the sensory experience of your meals. Mindful eating creates a healthy connection with food.

By combining these cooking methods and ideas into your culinary practices, you not only enhance the nutritional worth of your meals but also build a conscious and joyful attitude to eating. As you continue to explore protein-rich choices, remember that the path to an anti-inflammatory lifestyle is about balance, diversity, and the pleasure of fueling your body with nutritious, delectable meals. Let's begin on the next part of your culinary journey, appreciating the richness that protein-rich selections offer to your table and the good influence they have on your overall well-being.

Weeks 27-39: Flavorful Herbs & Spices

Chapter four

Anti-Inflammatory Herbs

Herbs not only add depth and complexity to foods but may also deliver a plethora of health advantages. Many herbs are renowned for their anti-inflammatory qualities, making them useful complements to an inflammation-reducing diet. Let's study a range of anti-inflammatory herbs and how to include them into your meals:

1. Turmeric:

Curcumin, the main ingredient in turmeric, is a strong anti-inflammatory drug.

Use turmeric in curries, soups, or
smoothies to leverage its health
advantages.

2. Ginger:
Ginger has significant
anti-inflammatory and antioxidant
properties. Incorporate fresh or ground
ginger into stir-fries, teas, or salad
dressings for a spicy kick.

3. Cinnamon:
- Cinnamon not only provides warmth
to foods but also has
anti-inflammatory qualities. Sprinkle
it over oatmeal, yogurt, or use it in
baking for a warming taste.

4. Rosemary:
 Rosemary includes rosmarinic acid, which has anti-inflammatory and antioxidant benefits. Use rosemary to flavor roasted vegetables, grilled meats, or in marinades.

5. Basil:
Basil is rich in chemicals like eugenol and linalool, recognized for their anti-inflammatory qualities. Add fresh basil to salads, spaghetti, or create a vivid pesto.

6. Oregano:
 Oregano includes carvacrol, a molecule having anti-inflammatory and antibacterial effects.

Use oregano in Mediterranean meals, soups, or sprinkle it over roasted veggies.

7. Thyme:
Thyme includes thymol, which has anti-inflammatory and antibacterial properties. Add thyme to roasted meats, stews, or use it in herb-infused oils.

8. Cilantro:
Cilantro is not just tasty but also includes antioxidants with possible anti-inflammatory properties. Include cilantro in salads, salsas, or garnish soups.

9. Sage:
Sage includes chemicals including rosmarinic acid and luteolin, adding to its anti-inflammatory benefits. Use sage in stuffing, pasta recipes, or as a flavor for roasted vegetables.

10. Mint:
Mint has cooling benefits and includes antioxidants that may have anti-inflammatory effects. Add fresh mint to salads, drinks, or use it in fruit-infused water.

Spice Blends for Health

Creating personal spice mixes enables you to adjust tastes to your preference while optimizing health benefits.

Spice blends not only add dimension to your foods but also deliver a concentrated dosage of numerous minerals and antioxidants. Here are some health-promoting spice combinations to enrich your culinary creations:

1. Golden Spice Blend:
Combine ground turmeric, ginger, cinnamon, and a pinch of black pepper. This mix is flexible and may be used in curries, soups, or sprinkled over roasted vegetables.

2. Mediterranean Herb Mix:
Mix dried oregano, thyme, rosemary, basil, and a pinch of garlic powder.

Use this combination in Mediterranean-inspired recipes, salads, or as a rub for grilled meats.

3. Cajun Spice Mix:
Create a Cajun mix using paprika, cayenne pepper, thyme, oregano, and garlic powder. Use it to season meats, roasted vegetables, or in rice recipes.

4. Chai Spice Blend:
Blend cinnamon, cardamom, ginger, cloves, and nutmeg for a warming chai spice blend. Add it to porridge, smoothies, or use it in baking for a comforting taste.

5. Herbes de Provence:
Combine dried rosemary, thyme,
oregano, lavender, and marjoram for a
traditional French herb combination.
Use it in roasted meals, soups, or as a
spice for grilled meats.

6. Harissa Spice Mix:
Create a spicy and tasty harissa mix
using ground cumin, coriander,
caraway seeds, smoked paprika, and
cayenne pepper. Use it as a rub or in
recipes for a powerful kick.

7. Italian Seasoning:
Mix dried basil, oregano, rosemary,
thyme, and garlic powder for an
Italian-inspired combination.

Sprinkle it over spaghetti, pizza, or use it in tomato-based recipes.

8. Curry Powder:
Blend powdered cumin, coriander, turmeric, ginger, and a dash of cayenne for a homemade curry powder. Use it in curries, lentil recipes, or to flavor rice.

9. Mexican Spice Mix:
 Combine chili powder, cumin, paprika, garlic powder, and oregano for a Mexican-inspired combination. Use it in tacos, enchiladas, or as a spice for grilled veggies.

10. Za'atar Blend:
Mix dried thyme, sumac, sesame seeds, and a touch of salt for a Middle Eastern za'atar mix. Sprinkle it over flatbreads, salads, or use it as a spice for roasted veggies.

Enhancing Flavor without Sacrificing Health

Balancing taste and health is an art in culinary experimentation. Fortunately, you may do both by adding thoughtful techniques into your cooking. Here are techniques to boost taste without losing health:

1. Citrus Zest:
Use citrus zest (lemon, lime, or orange) to add brightness and freshness to foods. Zest includes fragrant essential oils without the additional acidity of the juice, offering a blast of taste to salads, marinades, and desserts.

2. Infused Oils:
Create infused oils using herbs like rosemary, thyme, or garlic. These oils offer dimension to your cuisine without the need for excessive quantities of salt or bad fats.

3. Vinegar Varieties:
Experiment with various vinegar

varietals, such as balsamic, apple cider, or red wine vinegar. They offer acidity and depth to meals without depending on salt

4. Homemade Broths:
Prepare handmade broths using fragrant vegetables, herbs, and spices. This savory foundation improves the taste of soups, stews, and rice dishes without the need for excessive salt.

5. Umami-Rich Ingredients:
Incorporate umami-rich items like mushrooms, tomatoes, and soy sauce. Umami gives a delicious dimension to your foods, avoiding the need for excessive salt.

6. Fresh Herbs as Garnish:
Use fresh herbs as a final touch.
Sprinkle chopped cilantro, parsley, or
chives on top of your foods to give a
blast of flavor and visual appeal.

7. Roasting for Intensity:
Roasting enhances tastes and
caramelizes natural sugars. Roast
veggies, nuts, or spices before adding
them into your dishes for an added
layer of flavor.

8. Quality Ingredients:
Start with high-quality, fresh
ingredients. Fresh vegetables, herbs,
and spices provide more powerful

tastes, enabling you to depend less on extra seasonings.

9. Balancing Sweet and Savory:
Experiment with balancing sweet and savory flavors in your cuisine. A touch of sweetness from fruits or honey may compliment savory tastes, providing a pleasant taste profile.

10. Fresh Garlic and Onion:
Embrace the fragrant power of fresh garlic and onion. These essentials give a strong foundation taste for many meals, avoiding the need for excessive salt.

11. Grated Parmesan or Pecorino:
Use little quantities of grated
Parmesan or Pecorino cheese to lend a
burst of salty and savory flavors to
salads, pasta, or roasted vegetables.

12. Toasting Spices:
Toasting entire spices before grinding
releases their vital oils, increasing
their tastes. Incorporate freshly
ground, roasted spices into your dishes
for a strong flavor.

13. Freshly Ground Pepper:
Elevate your foods with freshly ground
black pepper. Its fragrant heat
accentuates the entire taste, letting
you to cut less on salt.

14. Dijon Mustard:
 Dijon mustard lends tanginess and depth to salads, marinades, and sauces. It's a versatile component that offers taste without additional salt.

15. Herb-Infused Vinegars:
Make herb-infused vinegars using combinations like tarragon and white wine vinegar or basil and balsamic vinegar. These infusions provide fresh tastes to salads and marinades.

16. Homemade Salsas and Chutneys:
Prepare homemade salsas or chutneys using fresh fruits,

vegetables, and herbs. These sauces
add layers of flavor to grilled meats,
seafood, or tacos.

17. Cocoa and Coffee in Savory Dishes:
Consider adding a dash of chocolate or
coffee to savory foods. These
components give richness and depth,
improving the variety of tastes.

18. Herbal Teas in Cooking:
 Experiment with herbal teas in
cookery. Infuse teas like chamomile,
mint, or lemongrass into broths,
sauces, or desserts for distinct and
delicate tastes.

19. Reducing Sodium Gradually:
Gradually minimize the quantity of
additional salt in your recipes. Your
taste receptors will change with time,
enabling you to enjoy the natural tastes
of foods.

20. Creative Use of Sweet Spices:
Explore inventive applications of sweet
spices like cinnamon, nutmeg, or
allspice in savory foods. These spices
may bring warmth and richness
without the need for excessive salt.

By combining these savory herbs, spice mixes, and mindful cooking habits, you can raise the taste of your meals while prioritizing your health. Embrace the richness of varied tastes, and allow your culinary creations become a celebration of both pleasure and well-being. As we continue on our tasty adventure, remember that each meal is a chance to fuel your body and pleasure your senses.

Weeks 40-52: Detoxification and Weight Management

Chapter five

Cleansing Foods and Beverages

Detoxification entails assisting the body's natural processes of removing toxins and boosting general well-being. Including cleaning foods and drinks in your diet may assist in this process. Let's investigate a number of possibilities that contribute to detoxification:

1. Hydration with Water:
Start the day with a glass of warm water with a touch of lemon. This helps jumpstart your metabolism and improves liver function.

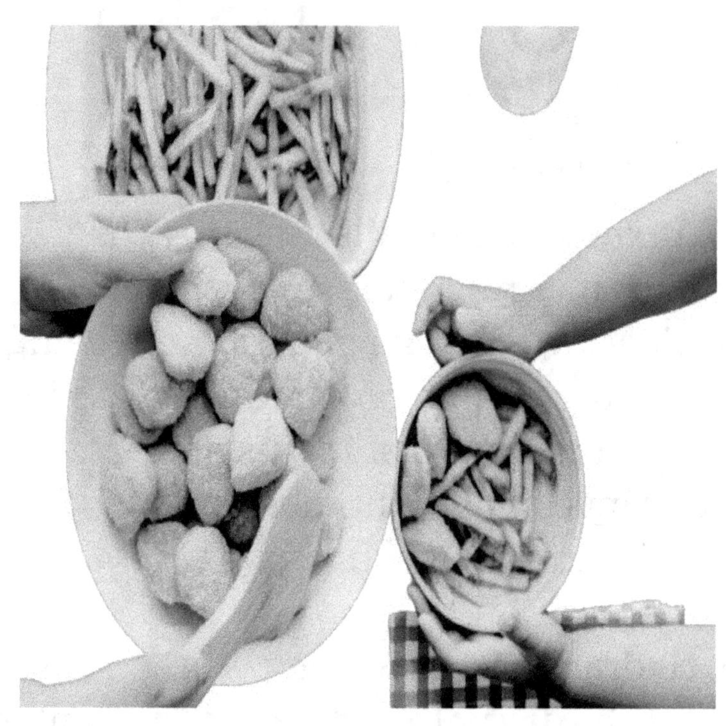

2. Green Tea:
Green tea is rich in antioxidants, notably catechins, which promote the body's detoxifying processes. Enjoy a cup in the morning or afternoon for a mild boost.

3. Detox Smoothies:
Create detox smoothies with ingredients like leafy greens, berries, cucumber, and aloe vera. These nutrient-packed drinks promote hydration and enhance overall wellness.

4. Citrus Fruits:
Citrus fruits including grapefruit, oranges, and lemons contain chemicals that stimulate liver detoxification. Incorporate them into your diet as snacks or in salads.

5. Leafy Greens:
Include leafy greens such as kale, spinach, and arugula in your meals. These veggies are high in chlorophyll, which promotes the body's detoxification functions.

6. Cruciferous Vegetables:
Broccoli, cauliflower, Brussels sprouts, and cabbage have chemicals that promote liver detoxification.

Enjoy them steaming, roasted, or in salads.

7. Beets:
Beets are known to promote liver function and aid with the removal of toxins. Roast or grate them for salads, or enjoy them in smoothies.

8. Turmeric:
 Turmeric includes curcumin, which has anti-inflammatory and antioxidant effects. Incorporate turmeric into your recipes or enjoy it in turmeric-infused drinks.

9. Herbal Detox Teas:
Explore herbal teas with detoxifying

plants including dandelion, milk
thistle, and burdock root. These teas
may be calming and supportive of liver
health.

10. Probiotic-Rich Foods:
 Include fermented foods like yogurt,
kefir, sauerkraut, and kimchi.
Probiotics maintain intestinal health,
which is crucial to total detoxification.

11. Detoxifying Herbs:
 Incorporate herbs like parsley,
cilantro, and mint into your meals.
These plants may aid in the removal of
heavy metals from the body.

12. Water-Rich Foods:
 Include water-rich meals like watermelon, cucumber, and celery. These foods help to hydration and assist the removal of pollutants.

13. Chia Seeds:
Chia seeds are high in fiber, which assists in digestion and the elimination of waste from the body. Add chia seeds to smoothies, yogurt, or overnight oats.

14. Activated Charcoal:
Activated charcoal may help absorb pollutants in the digestive system.

It's accessible in supplement form but should be taken carefully and under direction.

15. Alkaline Foods:
Choose alkaline-forming foods like leafy greens, almonds, and avocados. Alkaline diets are considered to promote the body's natural detoxification processes.

Practical Tips for Weight Loss

Maintaining a healthy weight is vital for general well-being. Here are practical ways to help weight reduction in a sustained and balanced way:

1. Mindful Eating:
Practice mindful eating by paying attention to hunger and fullness signs. Avoid distractions during meals and relish each mouthful.

2. Balanced Meals:
Create balanced meals that contain a combination of lean meats, complete grains, healthy fats, and lots of veggies. This helps keep you satiated and fulfills nutritional requirements.
3. meal Control: Be cautious of meal proportions to prevent overeating. Use smaller plates, and heed to your body's cues of fullness.

4. Regular Physical exercise:
Incorporate regular physical exercise
into your regimen. Find activities you
love, whether it's walking, cycling,
dancing, or yoga.

5. Hydration: Stay hydrated by
drinking water throughout the day.
Sometimes, sensations of hunger are
really indicators of dehydration.

6. Limit Processed Foods: Reduce the
consumption of processed and sugary
foods. Focus on full, nutrient-dense
meals that give lasting energy.

7. Meal Planning: Plan your meals and
snacks ahead of time.

This helps you make better decisions and prevent impulsive eating.

8. nutritious Snacking: Choose nutritious snacks like fresh fruit, almonds, or yogurt. Having healthful snacks on hand might avoid reaching for less healthy alternatives.

9. Quality Sleep: Prioritize quality sleep. Lack of sleep may alter hormones that control appetite and lead to cravings for high-calorie meals.

10. Stress Management: Find effective stress management strategies such as meditation,

deep breathing, or indulging in hobbies. Stress might lead to emotional eating.

11. Regular Meals: - Aim for regular and consistent meal times. This helps control hunger hormones and avoids excessive munching.

12. High-Fiber Foods: Include high-fiber foods including whole grains, legumes, fruits, and vegetables in your diet. Fiber increases satiety and intestinal health.

13. Lean Protein Sources: Choose lean protein sources such as chicken, fish, tofu, and lentils.

Protein is crucial for muscular health and helps you feel full.

14. Limit Liquid Calories: Be aware of liquid calories from sugary drinks and alcohol. Opt for water, herbal teas, or infused water for hydration.

15. incremental modifications: Make incremental modifications to your food and lifestyle. Sudden and abrupt adjustments are less likely to be sustainable in the long run.

Balancing Nutrient Intake

Balancing nutritional consumption is vital for general health and well-being.

Here are techniques to guarantee you're receiving a well-rounded assortment of nutrients:

1. Colorful Plate: Aim for a colorful plate by having a range of fruits and vegetables. Different hues signify specific minerals and antioxidants.

2. Whole Grains: Choose whole grains such as quinoa, brown rice, oats, and whole wheat. These grains include fiber, vitamins, and minerals.

3. Lean Proteins: Include lean protein sources such chicken, fish, eggs, tofu, and lentils. Protein is vital for muscle health and general bodily function.

4. Healthy Fats: Incorporate healthy fats from sources including avocados, nuts, seeds, and olive oil. These fats improve brain function and food absorption.

5. Dairy or Dairy substitutes: Include dairy or fortified dairy substitutes for calcium and vitamin D. These nutrients are necessary for bone health.

6. Variety of Vegetables: - Eat a variety of vegetables to guarantee a wide range of nutrients. Include leafy greens, cruciferous veggies, and colorful alternatives.

7. Fruits in Moderation: Enjoy a variety of fruits in moderation. While fruits give critical vitamins and antioxidants, be wary of natural sugars

8. Moderate Carb Intake: Choose carbs sensibly, focusing on complete, unprocessed choices. Whole grains, legumes, and starchy vegetables give sustained energy and important nutrients.

9. Nutrient-Dense Snacks: Opt for nutrient-dense snacks to suit your nutritional requirements between meals. Snack on veggies with hummus, Greek yogurt with berries, or a handful of almonds.

10. Adequate Hydration: Stay appropriately hydrated throughout the day. Water is needed for digestion, nutrition transfer, and general cellular function.

11. Vitamin-Rich Herbs: Incorporate vitamin-rich herbs like parsley and cilantro into your meals. These herbs not only offer taste but also supply critical nutrients.

12. Calcium-Rich Foods: Ensure you're receiving enough calcium from sources including dairy, fortified plant-based milk, tofu, and leafy greens.

13. Omega-3 Fatty Acids: Include
sources of omega-3 fatty acids, such as
fatty fish (salmon, mackerel),
flaxseeds, chia seeds, and walnuts.
These fats boost heart and brain
function.

14. Iron-Rich meals: Consume
iron-rich meals for good blood health.
Include lean meats, beans, dark leafy
greens, and fortified cereals.

15. Probiotic meals: Incorporate
probiotic-rich meals for gut health.
Yogurt, kefir, sauerkraut, and kimchi
are examples of fermented foods that
maintain a healthy microbiota.

16. Limit additional Sugars: Be aware of additional sugars in your diet. Choose whole fruits over sugary snacks, and check labels to find hidden sugars in processed foods.

17. Portion management for Balance: Practice portion management to promote a balanced intake of nutrients. Balancing your plate with adequate servings from various food categories helps overall wellness.

18. Rotate Protein Sources: – Rotate your protein sources to promote a broad amino acid composition. This not only helps to balanced nutrition but also offers variety to your meals.

19. Meal Diversity: - Aim for meal diversity by eating a combination of protein, carbs, healthy fats, and a range of veggies. This provides a wide variety of nutrients.

20. Regular Check-ins: Periodically review your nutritional intake and make modifications as required. Consider talking with a healthcare practitioner or qualified dietitian for individualized counsel.

Remember that establishing a balanced nutritional intake is a continuous process that incorporates individual requirements, preferences, and lifestyle circumstances. A broad and well-rounded diet offers the basis for general health and helps your path toward weight control and detoxification.

As you begin on the weeks devoted to detoxification and weight control, embrace these ideas as part of a comprehensive approach to well-being. By including cleansing meals, adopting practical strategies for weight reduction, and maintaining a balanced nutritional intake, you establish the framework for lasting health habits.

Each decision you make in your food and lifestyle journey adds to the vivid tapestry of your well-being. May this month be a time of nutrition, self-discovery, and the formation of habits that support your long-term health objectives.

Mindful Eating and Lifestyle Habits

Mindful Eating Practices

Mindful eating is a discipline that includes paying attention to the current moment while ingesting food. It stresses awareness of the sensory experience, ideas, and emotions linked with eating. Adopting mindful eating techniques may lead to a more balanced and joyful relationship with food. Here are crucial elements to add into your mindful eating journey:

1. Present Moment Awareness: Cultivate awareness of the present moment throughout eating. Engage your senses by savoring the colors, textures, and scents of your cuisine.

2. Slow and Savory Bites: Take your time to chew each mouthful fully. This not only assists digestion but also lets you to appreciate the tastes and textures of your meal.

3. Appreciation for components:
Develop an appreciation for the
components in your meals. Consider
the labor that went into planting,
harvesting, and cooking the food on
your plate.

4. thankfulness for sustenance:
Express thankfulness for the
sustenance your meal gives. Reflect on
the nutrients and energy that
contribute to your overall well-being.

5. Recognize Hunger and Fullness:
Tune in to your body's hunger and
fullness signals. Eat when you're
hungry and stop when you're content,
avoiding overeating.

6. Minimize Distractions: Create a focused dining environment by reducing distractions. Turn off technological gadgets, sit at a table, and concentrate on the act of eating without multitasking.

7. cautious Portioning: - Be cautious of portion amounts. Use smaller dishes and bowls, and heed to your body's cues to prevent mindless consuming.

8. Non-Judgmental Awareness: Approach eating with non-judgmental awareness. Release shame or judgment linked with dietary choices, establishing a healthy and balanced mentality.

9. Emotional Awareness: - Recognize emotional signs connected to eating. Be mindful of whether you're eating out of hunger, boredom, stress, or other emotions.

10. Mindful Snacking: - Extend mindful eating skills to snacks. Choose nutrient-dense snacks, and appreciate each mouthful with the same degree of attentiveness as a full meal.

11. Eating Rituals: Create rituals around eating. This might be reciting a quick grace, expressing appreciation, or just spending a minute of quiet before eating.

12. Experiment with Mindful Cooking: Extend attention to the cooking process. Pay attention to the scents, noises, and sensations involved in making your meals.

Stress Reduction Techniques
Managing stress is critical for general well-being, including having a good relationship with food. Chronic stress may lead to emotional eating and bad dietary choices. Incorporate these stress reduction tactics into your everyday life:

1. Deep Breathing techniques: Practice deep breathing techniques to elicit the relaxation response.

Inhale deeply with your nose, hold for a time, then exhale slowly through your mouth.

2. Mindful Meditation: Engage in mindful meditation to build a feeling of serenity and present awareness. Find a peaceful location, concentrate on your breath, and let go of rushing thoughts.

3. Progressive Muscle Relaxation: Systematically tension and then relax various muscle groups in your body. This method helps alleviate bodily tension linked with stress.

4. Nature Walks: Spend time in nature. Take slow walks in a park, forest, or other natural location to encourage relaxation and a connection with the environment.

5. Journaling: Keep a stress diary to reflect on your ideas and feelings. Writing may help you absorb stresses and uncover patterns in your reactions.

6. Mindful Movement (Yoga, Tai Chi): Engage in mindful movement techniques like yoga or Tai Chi. These practices blend physical activity with breath awareness, creating calm.

7. Digital Detox: Take vacations from digital gadgets. Limit screen usage, particularly before sleep, to decrease exposure to stress-inducing material.

8. Social ties: Foster social ties. Spend time with friends or family, discuss your ideas and emotions, and seek help at tough times.

9. Listening to peaceful Music: Create playlists of peaceful music. Listen to relaxing sounds to transform your attitude and create a serene environment.

10. Aromatherapy: Use essential oils or scented candles for aromatherapy. Scents including lavender, chamomile, and eucalyptus help encourage relaxation.

11. Boundary Setting: Set clear boundaries to control stresses. Learn to say no when necessary and prioritize self-care.

12. Laughter Therapy: - Incorporate comedy into your life. Watch a hilarious movie, attend a comedy concert, or indulge in activities that make you laugh.

13. Art and Creativity: Explore art and creative activities. Drawing, painting, or crafts may be soothing and give a creative outlet for stress reduction.

14. Gratitude Practice: Cultivate a gratitude practice. Regularly express thanks for good things of your life, establishing a happy outlook.

15. Massage or Self-Massage: Schedule a massage or practice self-massage methods. Massage helps remove bodily stress and promotes relaxation.

16. Warm Baths: Take warm baths with relaxing smells like lavender. This may be a pleasant and caring approach to unwind.

17. Progressive Goal Setting: Break down bigger activities into smaller, doable objectives. Celebrate modest victories along the way to alleviate stress associated to daunting undertakings.

18. Positive Affirmations: Use positive affirmations to improve your thinking. Repeat affirmations that resonate with you to foster a more optimistic mindset.

19. Mindful Eating as a Stress Reduction method: Practice mindful eating as a stress reduction method. Focus on the sensory sensation of eating to bring awareness to the current moment.

20. Professional help: Seek professional help if required. A therapist or counselor may give information and solutions for managing stress.

Incorporating Exercise for Overall Wellness

Regular physical exercise is crucial for total heath, including mental and emotional well-being. Exercise not only adds to physical health but also has tremendous benefits on mood and stress reduction. Here are methods to include fitness into your lifestyle:

1. Find Activities You like: Choose activities you actually like. Whether it's dancing, hiking, swimming, or cycling, picking activities you enjoy enhances the probability of persistent engagement.

2. Create a Routine:
Establish a regular workout program. Consistency is crucial, and having a regular routine makes it simpler to prioritize physical exercise.

3. Mix Cardio and Strength Training:
Incorporate a combination of cardiovascular and strength-training workouts. Cardio increases heart health, while strength training enhances muscular strength and metabolism.

4. start with Small Steps:
If you're new to fitness, start with simple,

manageable objectives. Gradually
increase intensity and duration as your
fitness level increases.

5. Outdoor Activities:
Take advantage of outdoor activities.
Outdoor exercise has the extra
advantage of exposure to nature, which
helps to mental well-being.

6. Group Classes or Sports:
Join group courses or engage in team
sports. Exercising with others may be
encouraging, and the social component
adds a fun element to your routine.

7. Home Workouts:
Incorporate home exercises into your schedule. There are countless internet tools, apps, and videos that give guided exercises for all fitness levels.
8. Mindful Movement Practices:
Engage in mindful movement methods like yoga or Pilates. These workouts not only enhance flexibility and strength but also encourage mental calm.

9. Interval Training:
Include interval training in your routines. Alternating between high-intensity and low-intensity

periods may enhance cardiovascular fitness and calorie burning.

10. Incorporate Movement Throughout the Day:
Find chances to exercise throughout the day. Take brief pauses to stretch, stroll, or conduct small activities to fight sedentary behavior.

11. Set Realistic Goals:
Set reasonable and attainable fitness objectives. Whether it's increasing daily steps, jogging a specific distance, or learning a new activity, having objectives keeps you motivated.

12. Variety in Workouts:
Keep your exercises varied to minimize boredom and target various muscle areas. Explore a range of activities to sustain interest.

13. Mind-Body Connection:
Cultivate a mind-body connection throughout exercising. Focus on how your body feels, your breathing, and the feelings of movement.

14. Prioritize Consistency Over Intensity:
Prioritize consistency above intensity. Regular, moderate exercise is more

sustainable and useful in the long term than irregular, hard exercises.

15. Include Flexibility Exercises:
Don't neglect flexibility exercises. Stretching or practices like yoga promote flexibility, alleviate muscular tension, and enhance general mobility.

16. Set a Positive Mindset:
Approach exercise with a good outlook. View it as a self-care exercise that adds to your entire well-being rather than a duty.

17. Mindful Walking or Running:
Practice attentive walking or running.
Pay attention to your surroundings,
the rhythm of your steps, and the sense
of movement.

18. Dance for Joy:
Incorporate dancing into your regimen.
Whether it's a dance lesson, dancing to
your favorite music at home, or
attending a dance fitness class,
dancing can be both enjoyable and a
fantastic exercise.

19. Choose Convenient Activities:
Choose activities that suit with your
lifestyle.

If time is a limitation, locate activities
that may be readily incorporated into
your regular routine.

20. Listen to Your Body:
Listen to your body and heed its cues. If
you need respite or a lesser exercise,
heed those requirements to avoid
burnout or damage.

21. Track Progress:
Track your progress. Whether it's
recording increases in strength,
endurance, or hitting fitness goals,
documenting progress helps enhance
motivation.

22. Mindful Cool Down:
Include a focused cool-down at the
conclusion of your exercises. Focus on
breathing and stretching to promote
relaxation and lessen post-exercise
stress.

23. Rest and Recovery:
Prioritize rest and recuperation. Your
body needs time to mend and adapt to
exercise. Ensure you allow yourself
appropriate sleep and recovery days
between intensive exercises.

24. Make it Enjoyable:
Make exercising pleasurable. Choose
hobbies that offer you delight,
 and don't hesitate to try new types of
physical exercise to keep things fresh.

25. Celebrate Achievements:
Celebrate your successes. Whether it's
accomplishing a fitness goal, learning
a new activity, or consistently adhering
to your regimen, appreciate your
efforts.

Incorporating mindful eating habits, stress reduction strategies, and regular exercise into your lifestyle promotes a holistic approach to well-being. Embrace these habits as interwoven components of a healthy and satisfying existence.

By nourishing your body and mind via mindful choices, you lay the road for prolonged health, resilience, and a healthy connection with yourself.

Seasonal Ingredients and Recipes

Embracing seasonal items in your cooking not only boosts taste but also assures that you're eating food at its freshest and most nutrient-rich form. Here are dishes featuring seasonal ingredients for each season:
Spring Recipes:

1. Strawberry Spinach Salad:
Ingredients:
Fresh spinach leaves
Sliced strawberries
Crumbled feta cheese
Toasted almonds
Balsamic vinaigrette
Instructions:
Toss together spinach, strawberries,
feta, and almonds.
Drizzle with balsamic vinaigrette
before serving.

2. Asparagus with Lemon Risotto:
1. ngredients:
Arborio rice
Asparagus spears, chopped

Lemon zest and juice
Vegetable broth
Parmesan cheese
instructions:
Sauté asparagus in olive oil.
Add rice, lemon zest, and gradually
whisk in broth until creamy.
Finish with Parmesan and a squeeze of
lemon.

3. Spring Vegetable Stir-Fry:
Ingredients:
Snap peas
Baby carrots
Broccoli florets
Bell peppers, thinly sliced
Tofu or chicken

Soy sauce with ginger
Instructions:
Stir-fry vegetables and protein in a wok
with soy sauce and ginger until
crisp-tender.

Summer Recipes:

1. Caprese Salad with Heirloom
Tomatoes:
Ingredients:
Heirloom tomatoes, sliced
Fresh mozzarella, sliced
Fresh basil leaves
Balsamic glaze
Olive oil, salt, and pepper

Instructions:
Arrange tomato and mozzarella slices.
Top with basil, drizzle with balsamic
glaze, olive oil, and season.

2. Grilled Corn and Avocado Salad:
Ingredients:
Grilled corn kernels
Diced avocado
Cherry tomatoes, halved
Red onion, finely chopped
Lime vinaigrette
Instructions:
Mix grilled corn, avocado, tomatoes,
and onion.
Toss with lime vinaigrette before
serving.

3. Lemon Garlic Shrimp Skewers:
Ingredients:
Large shrimp, peeled and deveined
Lemon juice with zest
Minced garlic
Olive oil
Fresh parsley, chopped
Instructions:
Marinate shrimp in lemon, garlic, and
olive oil.
Skewer and grill until done, decorate
with parsley.

Fall Recipes:

1. Butternut Squash Soup:
Ingredients:
Butternut squash, peeled and cubed

Onion, carrots, and celery
Vegetable broth
Coconut milk
Ground nutmeg and cinnamon
Instructions:
Sauté veggies, add broth, and simmer
until tender.
Blend, stir in coconut milk, nutmeg,
and cinnamon.

2. Apple Pecan Salad:
Ingredients:
Mixed greens
Sliced apples
Candied pecans
Blue cheese crumbles

Apple cider vinaigrette
Instructions:
Combine greens, apples, pecans, and blue cheese.
Drizzle with apple cider vinaigrette before serving.

3. Pumpkin Risotto:
Ingredients:
Arborio rice
Pumpkin puree
Sage leaves
Vegetable broth
Parmesan cheese
Instructions:
Sauté sage, add rice, and toss in pumpkin.

Gradually add broth until creamy, end
with Parmesan.

Winter Recipes:

1. Roasted Brussels Sprouts with
Cranberries:
Ingredients:
Brussels sprouts, half
Dried cranberries
Balsamic glaze
Olive oil, salt, and pepper
Instructions:
Toss Brussels sprouts and cranberries
in olive oil.
Roast till caramelized, sprinkle with
balsamic glaze.

2. Chicken and Vegetable Stew:
Ingredients:
Chicken thighs
Root veggies (carrots, potatoes)
Onion, garlic, and thyme
Chicken broth
Instructions:
Brown chicken, sauté veggies, add broth, and boil until cooked.

3. Quinoa Stuffed Acorn Squash:
Ingredients:
Acorn squash, half
Quinoa, cooked
Chickpeas, roasted
Pomegranate seeds
Maple tahini dressing
Instructions:

Roast squash, fill with quinoa,
chickpeas, and pomegranate.
Drizzle with maple tahini dressing.

Holiday and Celebration Modifications

Adapting recipes for holidays and
events helps you to preserve the festive
atmosphere while emphasizing health.
Here are tweaked renditions of
traditional favorites:

Healthier Thanksgiving Feast:

1. Herb-Roasted Turkey:
Use a blend of fresh herbs for seasoning
instead of excessive butter.
Roast turkey on a bed of veggies

including carrots, onions, and celery for extra taste.

2. Cauliflower Mash:
Replace regular mashed potatoes with cauliflower mash.
Steam cauliflower and combine with garlic, Greek yogurt, and a bit of Parmesan.

3. Quinoa with Cranberry Stuffing:
Substitute quinoa for conventional filling.
Mix quinoa with dried cranberries, chopped veggies, and herbs.

4. Roasted Brussels Sprouts:
Roast Brussels sprouts with a sprinkle
of balsamic glaze.
Add roasted almonds for crunch
instead of fried onions.

5. Sweet Potato Casserole:
Make a lighter sweet potato dish.
Mash sweet potatoes with a splash of
maple syrup, top with a nut and oat
crumble.

6. Lightened-Up Pumpkin Pie:
Use a whole grain crust or almond flour
crust.
Sweeten pumpkin pie filling using
natural sweeteners like maple syrup.

Healthy Dinner:

1. Baked Salmon:
Opt for baked salmon as a lean protein
alternative.
Marinate salmon with herbs, lemon,
and a dash of olive oil.

2. Quinoa and Vegetable Pilaf:
Replace heavy rice pilaf with quinoa.
Mix quinoa with sautéed veggies,
herbs, and a touch of lemon.

3. Green Bean Almondine:
Lighten up green beans almondine.

Steam green beans and combine with
toasted almonds, lemon, and a dab of
olive oil.

4. Herb-Roasted Potatoes:
Roast potatoes with herbs and a
minimum quantity of olive oil.
Include a variety of colored potatoes for
extra benefits.

5. Winter Fruit Salad:
Prepare a festive winter fruit salad.
Combine citrus segments,
pomegranate arils, kiwi slices, and
mint for a refreshing and colorful side.

6. Light Eggnog:
Create a lighter version of eggnog.
Use low-fat milk, Greek yogurt, and a
sprinkle of nutmeg for a creamy and
festive drink.

7. Vegetarian Wellington:
Opt for a vegetarian Wellington as a
centerpiece.
Wrap a combination of sautéed
mushrooms, spinach, and almonds in
puff pastry for a delicious and fulfilling
alternative.

8. Festive Fruit Sorbet:
Serve a cheerful fruit sorbet for dessert.

Blend frozen berries with a splash of lemon juice for a pleasant and guilt-free dessert.

New Year's Eve Appetizers:

1. Caprese Skewers:
Create bite-sized Caprese skewers using cherry tomatoes, fresh mozzarella, and basil.
Drizzle with a balsamic glaze for a punch of flavor.

2. Stuffed Mushrooms:
Prepare filled mushrooms with a combination of herbs, breadcrumbs, and a touch of olive oil.

Bake till golden for a delicious
appetizer.

3. Greek Yogurt Dip:
Make a healthy dip using Greek yogurt
as a basis.
Add herbs, garlic, and lemon for a
delicious dip served with vegetable
sticks.

4. Smoked Salmon Roll-Ups:
Roll smoked salmon with cream cheese
and dill for attractive and low-carb
canapés.

5. Roasted Vegetable Platter:
Roast a variety of colorful veggies and
serve with a mild dipping sauce.
Include bell peppers, zucchini, cherry
tomatoes, and asparagus.

6. Quinoa Stuffed Peppers:
Create small quinoa stuffed peppers as
a hearty and healthful treat.
Fill half peppers with a combination of
quinoa, black beans, corn, and
seasonings.

7. Fruit Salsa with Cinnamon Chips:
Prepare a fruit salsa using chopped
berries, kiwi, and mango.

Serve with homemade cinnamon chips prepared from whole grain tortillas.

8. Avocado Shrimp Cocktail:
Make a fresh avocado shrimp cocktail with poached shrimp, avocado cubes, and a zesty cocktail sauce.

Healthy Birthday Celebrations:

1. Whole Wheat Pizza with Veggie Toppings:
Opt for whole wheat pizza dough and fill it with colorful veggie toppings. Include bell peppers, tomatoes, spinach, and mushrooms for a nutritional variation.

2. Greek Salad Cups:
Serve Greek salad in separate cups for a
delicious and light snack.
Toss cucumber, cherry tomatoes,
olives, and feta with a lemon
vinaigrette.

3. Grilled Chicken Skewers:
Grill chicken skewers in a marinade of
lemon, garlic, and herbs.
Thread with cherry tomatoes and bell
peppers for a delicious and
protein-packed alternative.

4. Fruit Kabobs:
Create fruit kabobs using a selection of
fresh fruits.
Choose vibrant fruits like strawberries,
pineapple, grapes, and melon.

5. Quinoa Stuffed Bell Peppers:
Make quinoa stuffed bell peppers for a
substantial and healthful dinner meal.
Fill peppers with a combination of
quinoa, lean ground turkey, black
beans, and seasonings.

6. Dark Chocolate-Dipped
Strawberries:
Indulge in dark chocolate-dipped
strawberries for a delectable treat.

Dip fresh strawberries in melted dark chocolate and let them set.

7. Yogurt Parfait Bar:
Set up a yogurt parfait station with numerous toppings.
Offer alternatives like granola, almonds, fresh berries, and honey for a personalized dessert.

8. Vegetarian Spring Rolls:
Prepare vegetarian spring rolls using rice paper wrappers loaded with bright vegetables and tofu.
Serve with a mild peanut dipping sauce for extra taste.

Additionally, These seasonal and adapted recipes give a great selection of alternatives for a range of occasions. Whether you're embracing the tastes of each season or tweaking old favorites for holidays and festivals, these recipes promote health without sacrificing on pleasure. Enjoy the experience of discovering varied ingredients, attempting new culinary methods, and tasting the delectable outcomes as you make meals that feed both the body and the spirit.

Chapter six

Tips for Dining Out and Social Situations

Eating out and attending social events are vital components of life, and they typically entail navigating a range of food alternatives. Making healthy choices at restaurants, handling social settings, and striking a balance between fun and health are vital for overall well-being.

Here are guidelines to help you make thoughtful decisions in certain scenarios:

Making Healthy Choices at Restaurants:

1. Review the Menu Ahead of Time:
Before going to a restaurant, have a peek at the menu online. This helps you to make educated choices and avoid hasty selections based on hunger.

2. Choose Lean Protein Options:
Opt for lean protein sources such as grilled chicken, fish, or lentils. These alternatives give important nutrition without excessive saturated fats.

3. Embrace Vegetables and Salads:
Incorporate vegetables into your diet by picking salads, steaming, or roasted veggies. They provide fiber and vitamins to your dish.

4. Mindful Portion Control:
Be cautious about portion sizes. Consider splitting a meal with a friend or taking a bit home if portions are substantial.

5. Request Modifications:
 Don't hesitate to ask for alterations to fit your tastes or dietary restrictions. Restaurants typically accommodate requests for modifications.

6. Limit Liquid Calories:
Be wary of calorie-laden drinks. Opt
for water, herbal tea, or other
low-calorie choices instead of sugary
beverages.

7. Watch for Hidden Calories:
Be careful of hidden calories in
dressings, sauces, and condiments.
Ask for them on the side to restrict your
intake.

8. Savor Mindfully:
Eat gently and relish each mouthful.
This provides your body time to
communicate satiety, reducing
overeating.

9. Balance Your Plate:
Aim for a balanced dish with a mix of protein, healthy grains, and veggies. This guarantees a diversity of nutrients in your food.

10. Limit Fried and Processed Foods:
Minimize intake of fried and excessively processed meals. Opt for grilled, baked, or steaming alternatives.

11. Choose Whole Grains:
When feasible, pick whole grains over processed grains. Whole grains give greater fiber and minerals.

12. Practice Moderation with Treats:
If you desire a dessert, try sharing it with others to have a taste without overindulging.

3. Stay Hydrated:
Drink water during your meal. Staying hydrated promotes digestion and may help you notice actual hunger signals.

14. Be Mindful of Alcohol Intake:
Limit alcohol consumption. If you prefer to drink, do it in moderation and select lower-calorie choices.

15. Don't Skip Meals Beforehand:
Avoid missing meals before eating out.
This might lead to overeating owing to
increased appetite.

Navigating Social Gatherings:

1. Eat a Balanced Snack Beforehand:
Have a healthy snack before attending
social occasions to reduce severe
hunger and make better choices.

2. Contribute a Healthy Dish:
If appropriate, bring a nutritious meal
to share. This guarantees there's a
healthful choice accessible.

3. Survey the Spread:
Take a minute to explore the food alternatives before heaping your plate. Choose a range of products to make a balanced lunch.

4. Practice the 80/20 Rule:
Follow the 80/20 rule, opting for healthy choices 80% of the time and allowing for sweets at social events.

5. Engage in Conversation:
- Focus on participating in discussions rather focusing just on the food. This adjustment of concentration helps minimize mindless eating.

6. Use Smaller Plates:
If feasible, use a smaller plate to aid with portion control. It creates the appearance of a full plate with less food.

7. Stay Active During Socializing:
Engage in activities or games during social occasions to keep active. This may help balance the calories eaten.

8. Set Realistic Expectations:
 Set reasonable expectations for social occasions. It's alright to indulge sometimes, but strive for moderation.

9. Be Selective with Treats:
Be selective with sweets and desserts.
Choose the ones you actually appreciate
rather than simply trying everything.

10. Hydrate Between Alcoholic Drinks:
If drinking alcohol, alternate with
water between drinks to keep hydrated
and limit calorie intake.

11. Mindful Eating in Buffet Settings:
 In buffet situations, start with a
modest piece and go back for seconds if
required. This helps avoid overeating.

12. Focus on Quality, Not Quantity:
Focus on the quality of the meal rather
than quantity.

Enjoying lesser servings of high-quality food might be more rewarding.

13. Listen to Your Body:
Pay heed to your body's hunger and fullness signs. Stop eating when you're full, even if there's food remaining.

14. Plan Active Social Activities:
Plan social activities that require physical mobility, such as hiking, dancing, or playing sports.

15. Have a Support System:
Share your health objectives with friends or family to establish a support system.

Having individuals who understand your decisions might make socializing simpler.

Balancing Enjoyment and Health:

1. Embrace the 90/10 Lifestyle:
Adopt a 90/10 strategy, concentrating on making healthy choices most of the time while leaving flexibility for rare indulgences.

2. Practice Mindful Eating:
Embrace mindful eating concepts. Pay attention to tastes, sensations, and your body's cues to create a better connection with food.

3. Create Sustainable Habits:
Focus on building permanent habits
rather than short-term limits. This
adds to long-term health and
well-being.

4. Set Realistic Goals:
Set reasonable and attainable health
objectives. Celebrate minor triumphs
and progress toward a balanced
lifestyle.

5. Prioritize Enjoyable Activities:
Prioritize activities that offer pleasure
and satisfaction beyond eating. This
might include hobbies, socializing, or
physical activity.

6. Plan Treats Mindfully:
Plan treats carefully rather than responding to impulsive urges. Knowing when and why you indulge improves the delight.

7. Practice Intuitive Eating:
Explore intuitive eating, listening into your body's signals and eating in response to hunger and fullness.

8. Build a Positive Mindset:
Cultivate a good perspective about food and health. Avoid guilt connected with sweets and concentrate on feeding your body.

9. Explore New Healthy Recipes:
Make finding new, healthy recipes a
pleasant experience. Experimenting
with varied cuisines may make eating
healthy interesting.

10. Celebrate Non-Food Achievements:
Celebrate accomplishments that don't
center on eating. Acknowledge
personal progress, successes, and
milestones.

11. Practice Gratitude:
Cultivate thankfulness for the healthful
dietary options accessible to you. This
approach might boost the satisfaction
of eating properly.

12. Reflect on Food Choices:
Reflect on your eating choices without judgment. Understand the reasoning behind your decisions and make modifications as appropriate.

13. Establish a Routine:
Establishing a routine that corresponds with your health objectives might make it simpler to maintain a balance between fun and health. Consistency in eating times and selections develops a feeling of control.

14. Learn to Manage Stress:
 Stress may alter dietary choices. Develop effective stress management

skills such as meditation, deep breathing, or participating in activities that offer calm.

15. Seek Professional Guidance:
If required, connect with a qualified dietitian or nutritionist to obtain specialized counsel. They can help you build a balanced and sustainable eating plan.

16. Practice Resilience:
Approach obstacles with resilience. If you stray off track, acknowledge it as a short setback and concentrate on your health objectives.

17. Educate Yourself:
Stay educated about diet and health.
Understanding the advantages of
particular meals helps you to make
educated decisions.

18. Prioritize Sleep:
Quality sleep is vital for general
well-being, including keeping a
healthy balance in your eating choices.
Prioritize a regular and adequate sleep
pattern.

19. Include Enjoyable Physical
Activities:
Engage in physical activities you
actually like. Whether it's dancing,

hiking, or playing a sport, making exercise pleasant leads to a better lifestyle.

20. Connect with Like-Minded Individuals:
Surround yourself with folks who have similar health objectives. This supportive setting might make it simpler to make thoughtful decisions in many circumstances.

21. Explore Culinary Creativity:
Explore culinary creativity by testing various recipes and cooking techniques. This not only adds excitement to your meals but also encourages a broad and balanced diet.

22. Understand Emotional Eating:
Recognize emotional eating tendencies and treat the core reasons. Seeking other coping techniques helps avoid dependency on food for emotional comfort.

23. Practice Graciousness:
Be generous with yourself. Accept that perfection is unachievable, and occasional indulgences are part of a balanced approach to health.

24. Engage in Periodic Reflection:
Periodically reflect on your general well-being. Consider how your lifestyle,

including dietary choices, corresponds with your beliefs and long-term health objectives.

25. Celebrate Food Diversity: Embrace the variety of meals. Experiment with cuisines from many nations, including a diversity of tastes, spices, and ingredients into your meals.

26. Create a Supportive Environment: Shape your surroundings to support your health objectives. Stock your kitchen with nutritional alternatives, and surround yourself with good influences.

27. incorporate Mindful Cooking:
Engage in mindful cooking. Pay
attention to the process, relishing each
step, and appreciating the ingredients
you utilize.

28. Set Boundaries:
Establish limits around dietary choices
that match with your health aims.
Communicate these limits with people
close to you.
29. Dine with Purpose:
When eating out or socializing, have a
clear objective beyond merely the meal.
Whether it's enjoying the company,
commemorating an event,

or discovering new gastronomic sensations, concentrate on the greater context.

30. Celebrate Progress:
Celebrate your progress, no matter how tiny. Recognize the beneficial improvements you've made in your attitude to food and health.

In the path to balance fun and health, it's vital to approach each part with a feeling of mindfulness and self-compassion. By cultivating a good connection with food and making conscious choices, you can build a lifestyle that not only supports your

health objectives but also adds pleasure
and satisfaction to your entire
well–being.

Sustainability and Long-Term Wellness

Creating Lasting Habits:

1. Start Small:
Begin by introducing tiny, doable
adjustments into your routine. Gradual
alterations are more likely to develop
enduring habits.

2. Identify Triggers:
Recognize triggers that lead to harmful
behaviors. Understanding the core
issues helps you to handle them
effectively.

3. Set Realistic Goals:
Set reasonable and realistic objectives.
Goals that are excessively lofty might
be depressing, but modest triumphs
build confidence.

4. Establish a Routine:
 Build habits around a steady routine. A
well-defined timetable helps
incorporate healthy activities into your
everyday life.

5. Connect behaviors: Associate new behaviors with old ones. Pairing a new habit with an established routine makes it simpler to remember and implement.

6. Focus on Consistency: Prioritize consistency above perfection. Consistent, little efforts contribute more to long-term success than occasional great ones.

7. Celebrate Milestones: Celebrate milestones along the road.

Acknowledge and praise yourself for successes, building a positive relationship with healthy behaviors.

8. Adapt to obstacles: Anticipate obstacles and devise solutions to overcome them. Being adaptive in the face of adversity enables continuing advancement.

9. Create a Supportive atmosphere: Surround yourself with a supportive atmosphere. Ensure your environment encourage healthy choices and reward good actions.

10. Incorporate diversity: Introduce diversity into your routine. A diversified and entertaining approach stops habits from getting routine.

11. Reflect frequently: Reflect on your behaviors frequently. Assess what is functioning well and where tweaks may be required for continual development.

12. Understand motives: Understand your motives. Connecting with the causes underlying your behaviors enhances your commitment to long-term wellbeing.

Chapter seven

The Role of Anti-Inflammatory Diet in Long-Term Health:

1. Foundation for Sustainable Health: The anti-inflammatory diet serves as a foundation for sustainable health. Its emphasis on full, nutrient-dense meals matches with long-term health objectives.

2. Reducing Chronic Inflammation: Chronic inflammation is connected to several health concerns. The anti-inflammatory diet helps decrease inflammation, boosting general well-being.

3. Balancing Macronutrients: The diet promotes a balance of macronutrients, including healthy fats, lean proteins, and complex carbs. This equilibrium maintains sustained energy levels.

4. Rich in Antioxidants: Antioxidant-rich foods in the diet battle oxidative stress, protecting cells from harm.

This is vital for long-term cellular health.

5. Supporting Gut Health: A emphasis on fiber-rich diets and probiotics helps gut health. A healthy stomach is vital for nutrition absorption and general immunological function.

6. Managing Weight: - The anti-inflammatory diet assists to weight management. Maintaining a healthy weight is a vital element in avoiding different chronic illnesses.

7. Promoting Cardiovascular Health: -
Emphasizing heart-healthy foods, the
diet improves cardiovascular health.
This is critical for minimizing the risk
of heart-related disorders over time.

8. Preventing Age-Related illnesses:
The anti-inflammatory diet's influence
on inflammation and cellular health
may help to preventing age-related
illnesses, enhancing lifespan.

9. durable and pleasurable: - The diet's
focus on healthy, delicious meals
makes it durable and pleasurable for
long-term adherence.

It becomes a habit rather than a
temporary fix.

10. adjustable to varying Lifestyles: -
The anti-inflammatory diet is
adjustable to diverse lifestyles, making
it possible for people with varying
tastes and dietary demands.

11. Educating for Informed Choices: -
Understanding the concepts of the
anti-inflammatory diet helps people to
make informed choices about the foods
they eat, leading to lifetime health.

12. Long-Term illness Prevention: By treating inflammation and improving general health, the anti-inflammatory diet plays a role in long-term illness prevention, building a foundation for well-being.

Building a Supportive Community:

1. Share Goals with Others: Communicate your health goals with friends, family, or coworkers. Sharing objectives generates a supportive community engaged in your achievement.

2. Join Health and Wellness Groups: Participate in health and wellness groups or communities. Connecting with like-minded folks provides encouragement and shared experiences.

3. Encourage Open Communication: Create an atmosphere of open communication. Encourage talks about health objectives, problems, and triumphs within your community.

4. Organize Group Activities: - Organize group activities focusing on wellbeing. Group hikes, culinary lessons, or exercise programs reinforce the feeling of community.

5. Celebrate successes Together: –
Celebrate successes collectively.
Recognizing and appreciating one
other's accomplishments fosters a
happy and motivated culture.

6. Provide and Seek assistance: Offer
assistance to others in their wellness
journeys and seek help when required.
Mutual encouragement improves the
link throughout the community.

7. Share Resources and Information:
Share useful resources and
information. Whether it's articles,
recipes, or suggestions, contributing
to the community's knowledge base
promotes everyone's well–being.

8. Create Accountability relationships: Establish accountability relationships within the community. Having someone to discuss progress with adds a dimension of commitment.

9. Host Healthy Potlucks: Organize healthy potlucks where community members may exchange nutritious meals. This increases gastronomic variety and fosters social bonds.

10. Engage in Group Challenges: Engage in wellness challenges as a group. Whether it's a fitness challenge or a healthy eating challenge, friendly competition may be encouraging.

11. Utilize Social Media channels: –
Leverage social media channels to
engage with a bigger group. Online
communities give a venue for
continuing support and conversation.

12. Attend Wellness Events Together: –
Attend wellness events or courses
together. Participating in educational
and experiential activities promotes the
feeling of community.

13. Create a Positive atmosphere:
Foster a positive and inclusive
atmosphere. A supportive community
is founded on encouragement,
understanding, and acceptance.

14. Encourage Personal development: -
Support personal development within
the community. Acknowledge and
celebrate unique journeys, knowing
that wellbeing is a personal and
dynamic experience.

15. Offer Practical aid: Provide practical
aid when required. Whether it's
assisting with food planning, fitness
regimens, or managing health
difficulties, a helping hand improves
the community.

16. Establish Regular Check-Ins: - Set
up regular check-ins within the
community.

These may be virtual or in-person events where members exchange updates, objectives, and experiences.

17. Celebrate Community Milestones: Celebrate community milestonesAcknowledge and appreciate collaborative accomplishments within the community. Milestones might include accomplishing a physical goal, adopting a new healthy habit, or completing a wellness challenge together.

18. Promote Inclusivity: Ensure that the community is inclusive and varied. Embrace diversity and create an atmosphere where everyone feels welcome and supported.

19. Provide Emotional Support: Offer emotional support during hard situations. Knowing that there's a community to draw on may be crucial in conquering problems.

20. Share Inspirational tales: Share inspirational tales within the community.

Personal accounts of change and perseverance inspire others and develop a culture of encouragement.

21. Collaborate on Wellness Initiatives: Collaborate on wellness initiatives. Whether it's creating a neighborhood fitness event or teaming for a nutrition course, coordinated efforts enhance the effect.

22. Encourage Lifelong Learning: Encourage lifelong learning within the community. Stay interested about new health trends, recipes, and wellness practices, encouraging a culture of continual development.

23. Host Guest lecturers: Invite guest lecturers or specialists to share ideas with the community. Learning from specialists gives richness to the collective knowledge of health and wellbeing.

24. Establish a communal Garden: Consider developing a communal garden. Growing and sharing fresh food develops bonds and encourages a shared commitment to good eating.

25. Offer Mentorship Opportunities: Create mentorship opportunities within the community. Those who have successfully incorporated healthy behaviors may advise and help others on their travels.

26. Organize Fitness Challenges: Organize fitness challenges or activities that members may engage in together. Friendly rivalry and shared successes improve the feeling of community.

27. Celebrate Cultural variety:
Acknowledge and celebrate cultural
variety within the community.
Recognizing varied viewpoints on

health strengthens the communal
experience.

28. Implement Peer Support Programs:
Establish peer support programs.
Pairing community members with
similar interests or difficulties develops
a network of mutual support.

29. Create Virtual Accountability
Groups: Facilitate virtual accountability
groups. Online platforms give
possibilities for members to
communicate, discuss progress, and
provide encouragement.

30. maintain communal Rituals:
Develop and maintain communal
rituals. Whether it's a monthly

wellness group or an annual health fair,
regular activities contribute to
community cohesiveness.

Building a supportive group serves a crucial role in preserving long-term wellbeing. By building relationships, sharing experiences, and collectively working towards health objectives, the community becomes a source of inspiration, motivation, and resilience for each member.

Conclusion

In conclusion, the route towards sustainability and long-term wellbeing entails forming enduring habits, recognizing the importance of an anti-inflammatory diet in general health, and cultivating a supportive network. Embracing tiny, regular adjustments, connecting with the concepts of a health-focused diet, and creating a network of support contribute to a holistic approach to well-being. As people and communities seek for longevity and vitality, the combination of personal dedication, educated decisions, and social support builds the basis for a healthy and lasting wellness lifestyle.